These Facts can make you Healthier

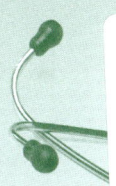

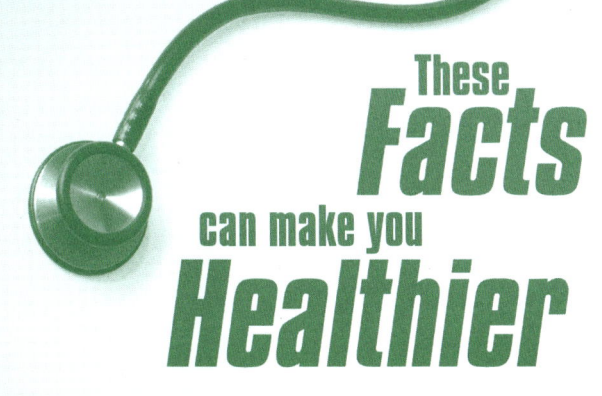

R. J. B. Willis

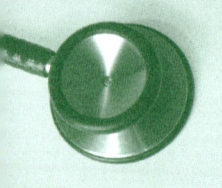

First published in 2010
Copyright © 2010 Autumn House (Europe) Ltd
All rights reserved. No part of this publication may be reproduced in any form without prior permission from the publishers.

British Library Cataloguing in Publication Data. A catalogue record for this book is available from the British Library.

ISBN 978-1-906381-74-5

Published by Autumn House (Europe) Ltd, Grantham, Lincolnshire.

Designed by Abigail Murphy.

Printed in Thailand.

Health is . . .

'Public health is the science and art of promoting health. It does so based on the understanding that health is a process engaging social, mental, spiritual and physical well-being. It bases its actions on the knowledge that health is a fundamental resource to the individual, the community and to society as a whole and must be supported through sound investments into conditions of living that create, maintain and protect health.'

Dr Ilona Kickbusch

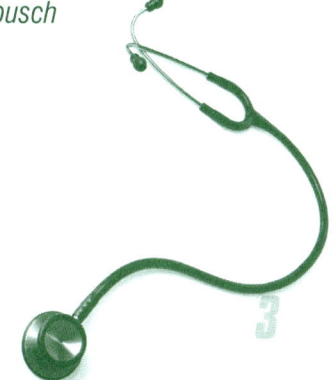

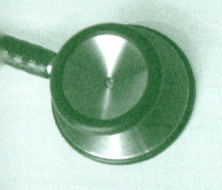

'Health is a large word. It embraces not the body only, but the mind and spirit as well; ... and not today's pain or pleasure alone, but the whole being and outlook of a man.'

James H. West

Hypochondria

'It is a most extraordinary thing, but I never read a patent medicine advertisement without being impelled to the conclusion that I am suffering from the particular disease therein dealt with in its most virulent form.'

Jerome K. Jerome

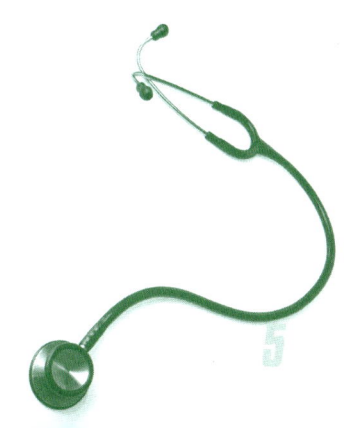

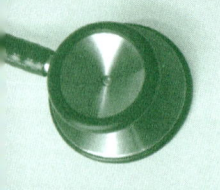

Pills – the answer to everything?

'I will lift mine eyes unto the pills. Almost everyone takes them, from the humble aspirin to the multi-coloured, king-sized three deckers, which put you to sleep, wake you up, stimulate and soothe you all in one. It is an age of pills.'

Malcolm Muggeridge

Pill-judged?

'A man's health can be judged by which he takes two at a time – pills or stairs.'
Joan Welsh

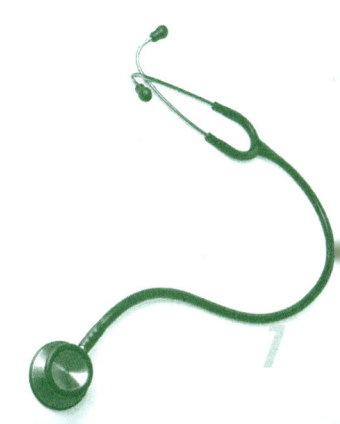

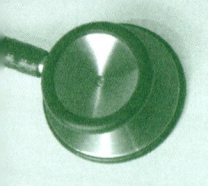

Decisions, decisions

'The longer I practise medicine, the more convinced I am there are only two types of cases: those that involve taking the trousers off and those that don't.'

Alan Bennett

Well, maybe!

A recent health enquiry concluded with the words, '. . . I want to have the benefits of good nutrition but I am disinclined to fuss about my food.' Much like the literary character, Sir Nicholas Gimcrack, who went around carrying out frog-like swimming motions. When asked what he was doing, he said that he was engaged in speculative swimming which was enough for him since he had no intention of taking to the water!

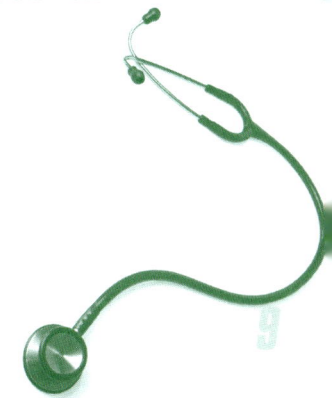

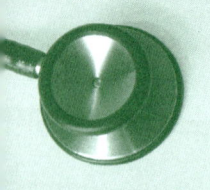

A little bit further

'Knowing is not enough, we must apply;
willing is not enough, we must act.'
Goethe

That's us!

Scientists have long dreamt of making a self-balancing, twenty-eight-jointed adapter-base biped, containing an electro-chemical reduction plant, with thousands of hydraulic and pneumatic pumps, with motors attached.

Such a being would have some sixty-two thousand miles of capillaries, millions of warning, railroad and conveyor systems, crushers and cranes, and having a universally distributed telephone system.

'. . . all that makes man'
(Tennyson).

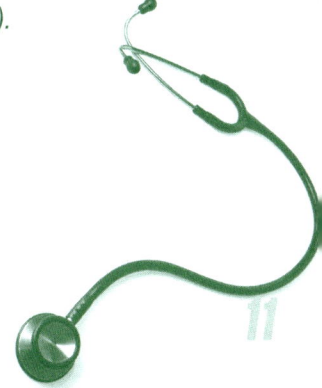

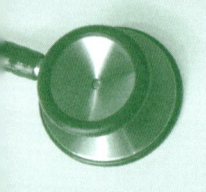

Health literacy

The US Surgeon General stated: 'Health literacy is the currency of success for everything we do in primary and preventive medicine.'

Health literacy refers to the skills of understanding and using health information, both written and verbal. Without these skills, health inequalities will widen and patient empowerment will fail.

WHO says . . .

The World Health Organisation says:
- 4.9 million people will die from tobacco use;
- 2.6 million will die from overweight and obesity;
- 4.4 million will die of raised cholesterol levels;
- 7.1 million will die of raised blood pressure;
- 388 million will die of chronic disease in the next decade (because of unhealthy diets, physical inactivity and tobacco use).

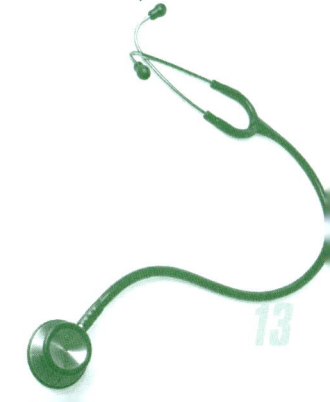

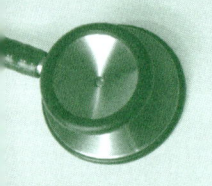

WHO aims . . .

. . . to get a 2% reduction in chronic disease death rates per year over the next decade.

It is estimated that this will prevent 36 million premature deaths by 2015.

Womb with a view!

'The health we enjoy throughout our lives is determined to a large extent by the conditions in which we developed in the womb. How we are ushered into life is the major factor that determines how we leave it. The quality of life in the womb, our temporary home before we were born, programmes our susceptibility to coronary artery disease, stroke, diabetes, obesity and a multitude of other conditions in later life.'

Professor Peter Nathanielsz

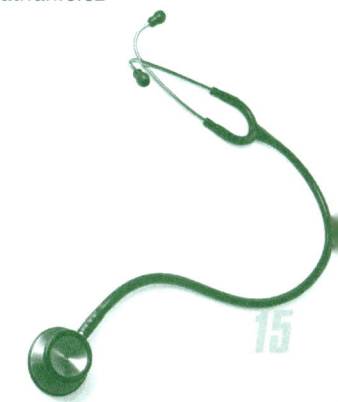

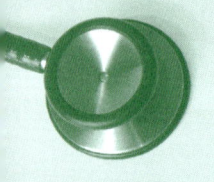

Male children born to mothers:
- exposed to starvation measures in the first third of their pregnancy had a greater tendency to obesity later in life
- starved in the final trimester of pregnancy had a decreased likelihood of later obesity

Nanny knows best

'Whatever is done for men or classes, to a certain extent takes away the stimulus and necessity of doing for themselves; and where men are subjected to over-guidance and over-government, the inevitable tendency is to render them comparatively helpless.'

Samuel Smiles (1859)

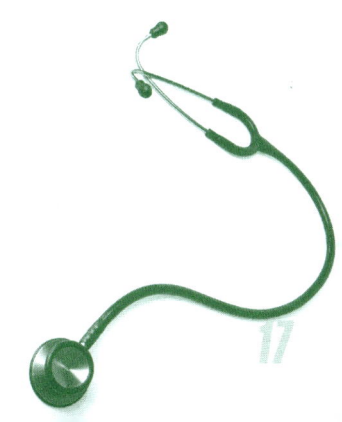

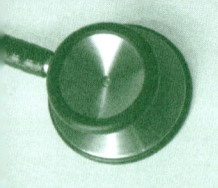

The middle path

'If you want people to choose a healthy lifestyle,
if you want people to give up smoking,
then you make them middle class.'

Dr John Reid, former UK Health secretary

Habit vs necessity

'Our habits commonly begin as pleasures in which we have no need and end as necessities in which we have no pleasure. Nevertheless we tend to resent the suggestion that anyone should try to change them, even on the disarming grounds that they do so for our own good. . . .

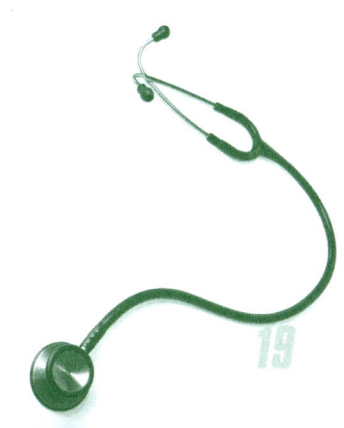

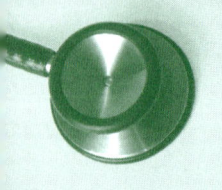

> '... It is said that the individual must be free to choose whether he wishes to smoke. But he is not free; with a drug of addiction the option is open only at the beginning, so that the critical decision to smoke is taken, not by consenting adults but by children below the age of consent.'
>
> *Thomas McKeown*

Dying to work

Although we know that smoking kills, we still allow over two million people in the UK to work in smoke-filled premises, and another ten million (38% of the workforce) to be exposed to cigarette smoke somewhere on the premises. Second-hand (passive) smoke in the workplace is estimated to kill 700 people a year, three times the number killed in industrial accidents.

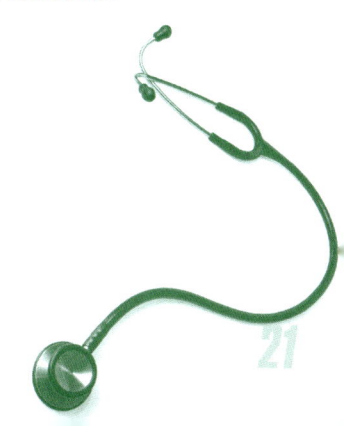

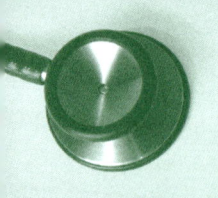

The smoking parrot

Or the choking parrot. A couple who spent more than £600 at the vets for antibiotics, allergy tests and nebulisers because their bird's beak ran and he sneezed all day have got to the root of the problem. Their smoking! For twenty years Jay Jay the Amazonian parrot had been passive smoking.

Playing with fire

'The sheer scale of damage that smoking causes to reproductive and child health is shocking.'

Dr Vivienne Nathanson

- 120,000 UK men aged 30-50 are impotent as a result of smoking
- smoking reduces pregnancy chances by up to 40% per cycle

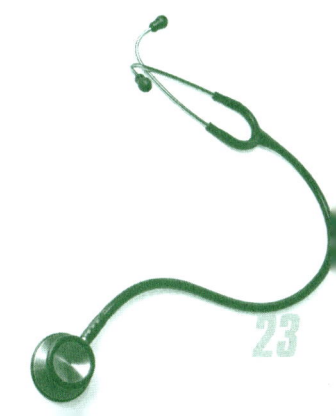

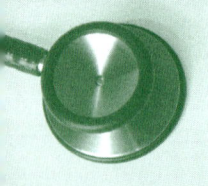

A captive audience

- Passive smoking has been linked to:
  * premature death
  * cot death
  * child respiratory problems
  * childhood asthma
- Around 17,000 children under age 5 in the UK are admitted to hospital each year due to passive smoking
- Women who smoke yield smaller volumes and decreased quality breast milk

Nicotine carriers

A Swedish study has found that the children of parents who smoke, even if outdoors with the door closed, had twice as much nicotine residue in their bodies as children of non-smokers.

If the parents had smoked indoors, the residue (*cotinine*) would have been fifteen times higher than children from non-smoking homes.

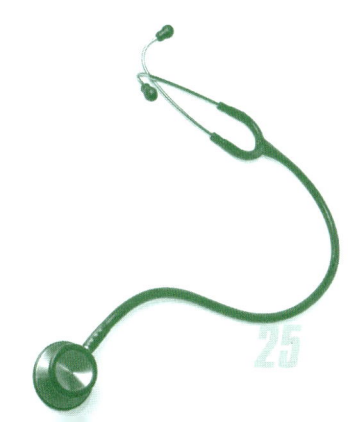

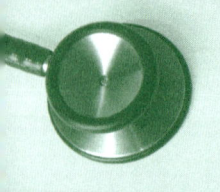

A change of heart

The advent of heart transplants has shed new and surprising light on the neuronal pathways involved in emotion and memory. A trickle of anecdotal accounts of memory changes in heart transplant patients has led to a relatively new field of research – *neurocardiology*.

When a heart is transplanted the nerve fibres are severed and may never reconnect, hence the possibility that memories are inherited via the transplant.

Heart to heart

Research shows that the heart has a 'brain' of its own. There are about 40,000 neurons – *sensory neurites* – in the heart's nervous system detecting circulating hormones, neurochemicals, heart-rate and pressure information which influence perception, decision-making and other cognitive processes.

The heart's own particular logic can override the data from the autonomic nervous system, thus causing the brain to 'obey' the heart and affect the individual's behaviour.

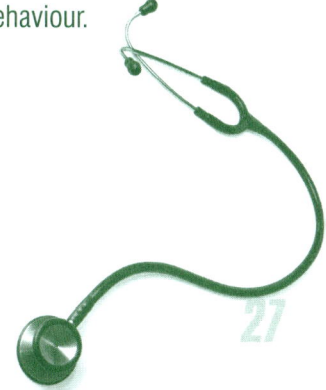

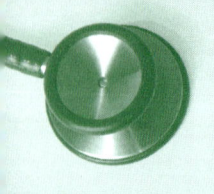

A hole (or two) in the heart

A new method has been proposed to restore blood flow to damaged hearts. It involves using a laser to cut a number of fine holes in the heart muscle having a reduced supply of blood. It is expected that the tiny holes will fill up with blood and stimulate new blood vessel growth.

Keeping pace

A team at the University of Colorado has introduced a new pacemaker, reducing the likelihood of death from heart rhythm disturbance by up to 36%. Costing around £20,000 per device, the pacemaker implanted under the left shoulder resynchronises the heart rhythms.

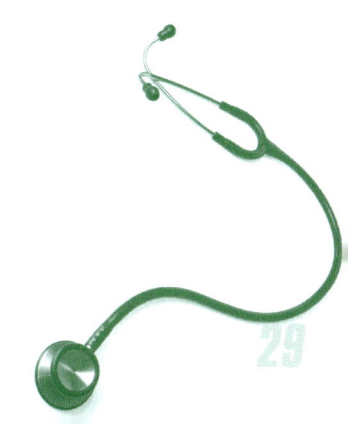

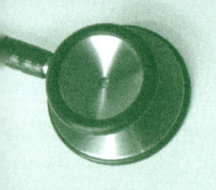

Heart'sease

A Manchester Royal Infirmary study concluded that having a very close relationship with a significant other person could up to halve a recurrence of heart attack.

WHO and mental health

According to the World Health Organisation, mental health is:

'a state of well-being in which the individual realises his or her abilities, can cope with the normal stresses of life, can work productively and fruitfully, and is able to make a contribution to his or her community.'

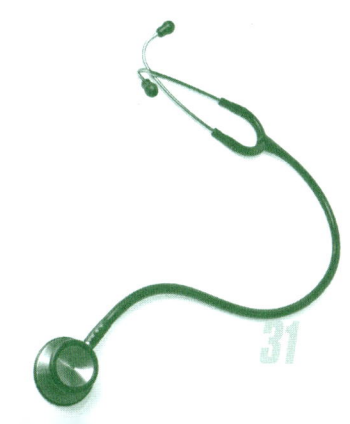

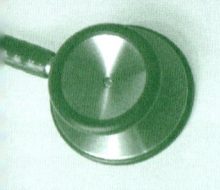

Mind: what you eat

'The time is now right for nutrition to become a mainstream, everyday component of mental health care, and a regular factor in mental health promotion.'

*Dr Andrew McCulloch, CE,
The Mental Health Foundation*

Talking to oneself

Brain research using the various new imaging devices and the monitoring of skin conductivity has highlighted the conclusion that voice hearers are literally speaking to themselves.

When the voices are heard activity can be found in both *Wernicke's* and *Broca's* areas of the brain, the regions that deal with speech. The muscles used in normal talking are also activated.

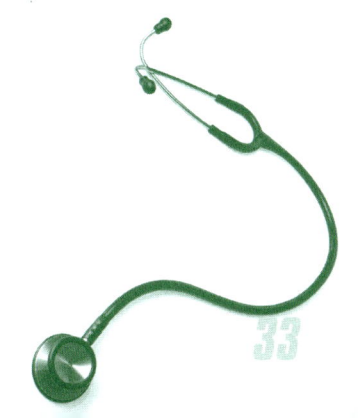

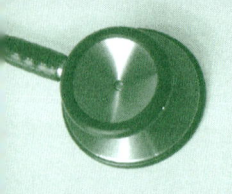

The inner speech silence and minuscule muscular activity is referred to as *subvocalisation*. It is thought to be a learned behaviour in that children talk to themselves out loud in early childhood, and then suppress the activity as they get older.

Even then, some older people vocalise their activities and often speak of 'thinking aloud'.

Blue genes

Research at the University of Pittsburgh discovered that a mutation of gene *CREB1* causes severe depression in women.

The interaction of the gene with the female hormone oestrogen is the likely cause of the depression. Animal studies show the exact amount of *CREB1* present is co-related to depression rates.

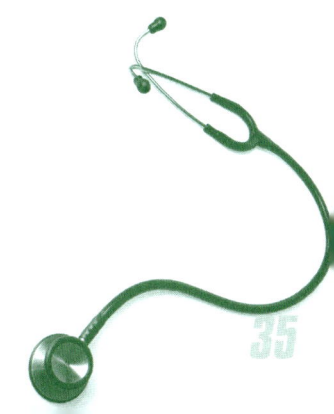

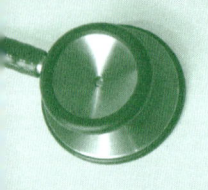

Too sad

A recognised cause of depression is Seasonal Affective Disorder (*SAD*). It appears to a condition in which the body clock is maladjusted by the rise and fall of *melatonin*, a secretion of the pineal gland in the brain.

Persons affected become depressed, listless, chronically fatigued and deeply moody.

The condition is virtually unknown in people living below the 30th parallel.

Li-li-like ttthis or . . . !?

Approximately 1% of the population has a stammer or a stutter. Around 2,936,554 (US), 325,078 (Canada), 602,707 (UK, with 29,180 in Wales).

The title depicts all three types of stuttering:

- **repetitions** *li-li-like* this
- **prolongation** like *ttthis*
- **abnormal stoppages** like . . .

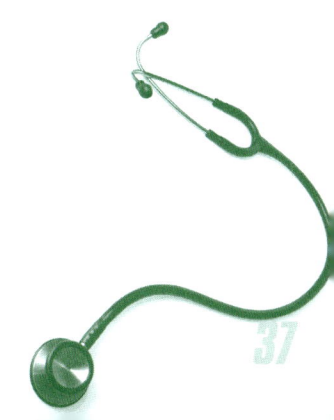

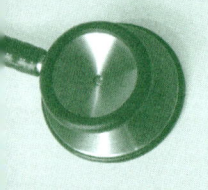

Four factors contribute to the development of stuttering:
- **genetics** (60% have a family history)
- **difficulties in child development** (speech or language difficulties or delays)
- **neurophysiology** (stutterers use different parts of the brain from non-stutterers)
- **lifestyle** (high family expectations and fast-paced lifestyles)

Name your poison

People who smoke and drink will not have to decide whether to buy cigarettes or beer in the future. A new beer – *Nicoshot* – combines alcohol and nicotine in one brew.

The German beer contains 3mgs of nicotine. Three cans of the beer have about the same nicotine content as a twenty-pack of cigarettes.

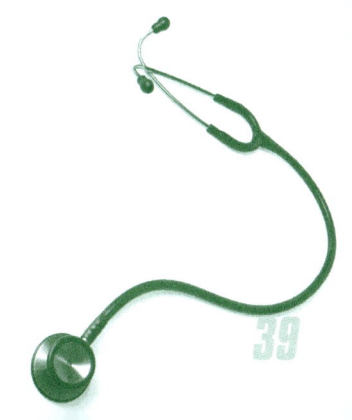

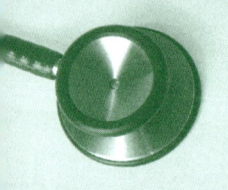

Chuckle count

Your daily laugh total should equal fifteen chuckles a day or you are underlaughed.

Dr Joan Gomez says, 'Stress is just part of everyday living for most of us. But there are ways of coping with it successfully. One of the best medicines is laughter. Laughter melts away stress like ice under a blow lamp.'

Chuckle muscles

Research into the effects of laughter – gelotology – shows that it increases the pleasure hormones (*endorphins*), which in turn increase the volume of oxygen in the blood, speed the heart rate, decrease blood pressure and relax the arteries. It is also a free treatment which can be used anywhere.

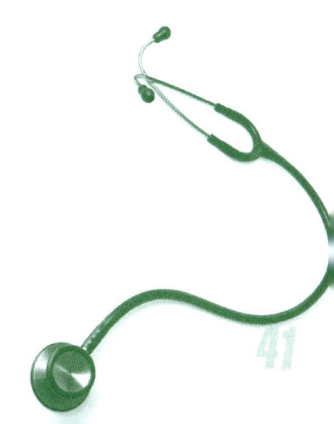

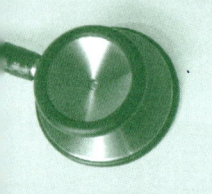

Red-nose day

A group of New York hospitals have a team of thirty-five clowns – the *Big Apple Circus* – which has been visiting the wards for nearly two decades.

Now the clinical vocabulary of the children's ward has changed. The children like the 'Kitty CAT scans', 'chocolate-milk transfusions' and 'red-nose transplants', thus alleviating their fear of the real thing.

'It may be possible to incorporate laugher into daily activities, just as is done with other heart-healthy activities, such as taking the stairs instead of the elevator. The recommendation for a healthy heart may one day be exercise, eat right and laugh a few times a day.'

*Michael Miller, MD, FACC,
Center for Preventive Cardiology at
the University of Maryland Medical Center*

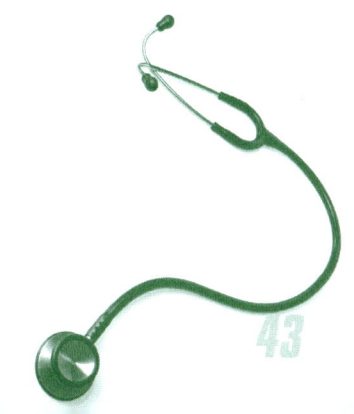

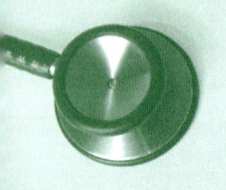

A singing heart?

'It is essential to our well-being, and to our lives, that we play and enjoy life. Every single day do something that makes your heart sing.'

Marcia Wielder

Doctor's orders

'After these two, Dr Diet and Dr Quiet,
Dr Merriman is requisite to preserve health.'
James Howell

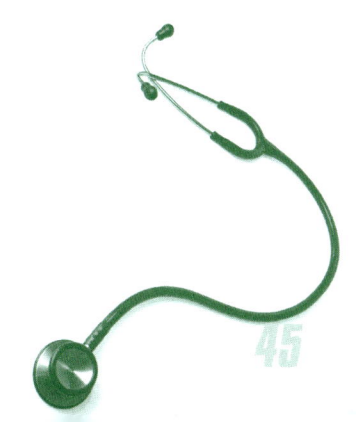

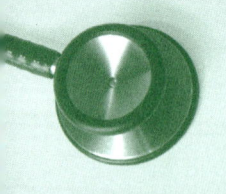

Witzelsucht!

Witzelsucht is the name given to pathologically misplaced humour (F. O. Witzel, 1856-1925). There are some people who feel uncontrollable laughter coming on in the most inappropriate places (funerals or other serious situations).

They have small lesions in the frontal lobes of their brains. Larger lobal damage can cause individuals to perform poorly on verbal jokes and miss humour in non-verbal cartoons.

Air traffic control

Asthma is a condition affecting the airways with the small tubes of the lungs becoming sensitive and inflamed.

Various irritants contribute to the condition, making the tubes narrower and thus harder to breathe.

The muscles controlling the breathing tighten, and the inflamed linings of the airways start to swell and produce sticky mucus or phlegm.

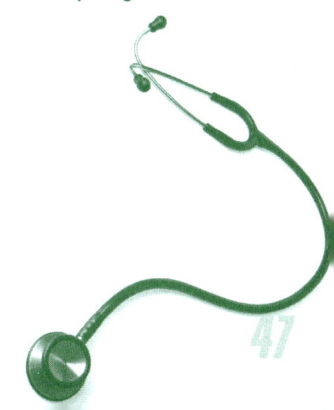

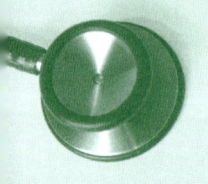

Asthma triggers

- flu illness early in life
- exposure to industrial and/or domestic cleaning agents
- vehicle exhaust fumes
- *nitro trichloride* (the by-product of pool chlorine, sweat and urine) in indoor pools
- early antibiotic use
- tobacco smoke
- house-dust mites
- mould spores and pollen
- pets

In praise of fleas!

Herman Melville (1819-91) was probably right when he said, 'No great and enduring volume can ever be written on the flea.' However, cadging a lift on a dog's back and being reviled by humans may be past for *Pulex irritans*. The flea has donated its body to science and may even have answered the poet Yeats' question: 'Was there ever a dog that praised his fleas?'

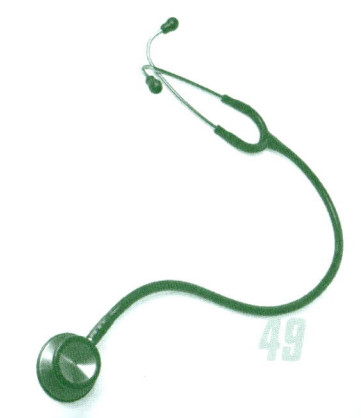

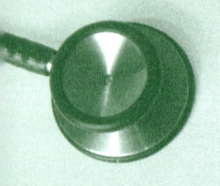

One short hop!

Australian researchers have discovered that a protein – *resilin* – responsible for the flea's ability to jump can be used to repair damaged arteries.

Resilin out-performs the highest grade rubbers available and is able to withstand the stresses placed on it and returns to its normal shape.

Artificial *resilin* can be used to restore the elasticity of arteries.

Down on the beach

'The South Beach Diet is pitched as being more moderate, easier to follow and safer than Atkins, but from what I can tell, the weight-loss "wolf" has just put on a different set of sheep's clothing.'

Professor T. Colin Campbell

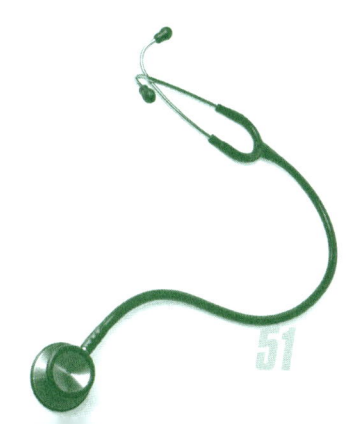

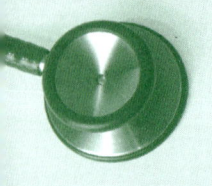

During the first six months of Atkins or South Beach dieting subjects have reported:
- constipation
- bad breath
- headaches
- hair loss
- increased menstrual bleeding

Children have experienced:
- calcium oxalate/urate kidney stones
- vomiting
- missed periods
- high cholesterol
- vitamin deficiencies

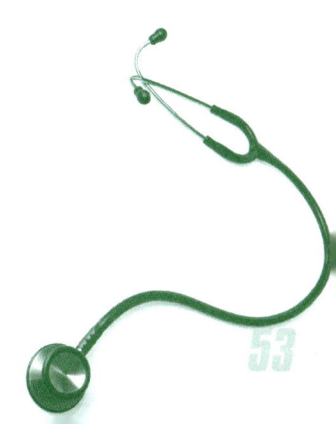

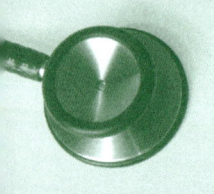

The nut behind the wheel

The most important part of a car is the nut behind the wheel! EU health leaders aim to safeguard the European roads from well-oiled nuts by introducing:

- a maximum blood alcohol concentration limit of 0.5g/l and breath equivalent throughout Europe
- a lower limit of 0.2g/l for novice drivers and drivers of public service and heavy goods vehicles

Dial-a-drunk

Telecommunications experts in South Korea have invented a telephone – dubbed the sobriety phone – that can detect whether or not the user is under the influence of alcohol. It has a built-in breathalyser. If the individual is well oiled, the phone screen displays a picture of a swerving car and can also prevent drunk dialling.

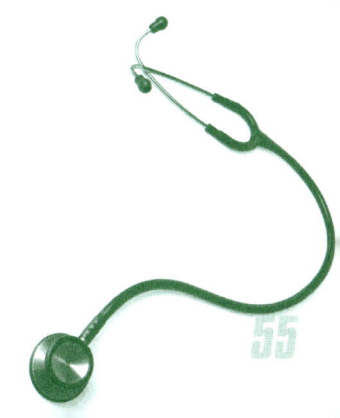

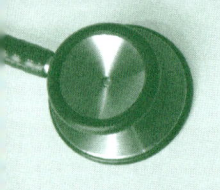

Moo Joose!

An Australian company (Wicked Holdings Pty Ltd) is trying to bring out a new drink for young people – *Moo Joose.*

The drink is a skimmed milk and 5.3% alcohol mixture with milkshake flavours: banana (Banana Smash); chocolate; coffee; and strawberry (Strawberry Rush).

As prescribed

'The desire to take medicine is perhaps the greatest feature which distinguishes man from animals.'
Sir William Osler (1849-1919)

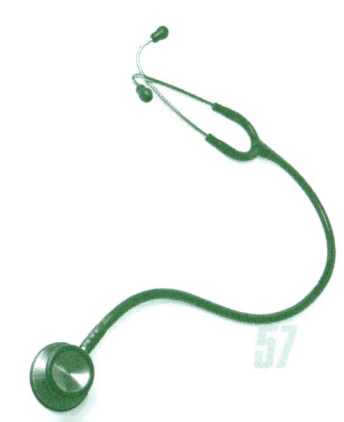

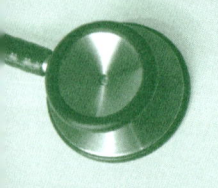

Faking it

According to WHO around 10% of *all* the drugs on sale globally are counterfeits.

Since various companies sell generic versions of named drugs in a variety of packaging these could turn up anywhere for sale.

The counterfeits are not necessarily of known drugs; they may be of completely inert substances.

Junk science

Korea's Woo Suk Hwang has put the scientific world into a state of chaos. His research towards 'therapeutic cloning' has been proven to be fabricated material.

Stem-cell research was thought to be making great strides with the many papers that he had published. He now faces criminal charges.

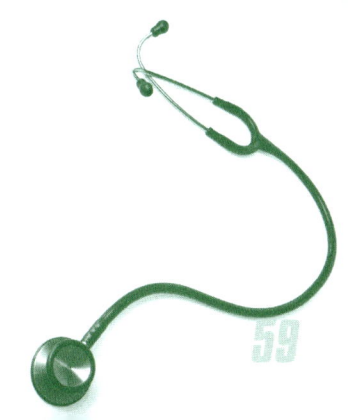

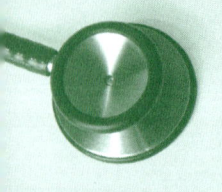

Caught by the hair

Hair extensions saturated with a solution of cocaine is new way of smuggling drugs. The *devil's dandruff* is washed out of the hair and re-crystallised for re-sale. The hair pieces present a challenge to drug detection as traffickers become more ingenious with their smuggling tactics.

Keeping kids safe

Modelling a healthy lifestyle will not guarantee that your child will be healthy, but the three leading causes of preventable death are already well started before young adulthood.

A project involving 14,000 young adults from early adolescence showed that diet, obesity, physical activity levels, tobacco, alcohol and illicit drug use, health care access, and acquiring a sexually transmitted disease worsened with the approach to adulthood.

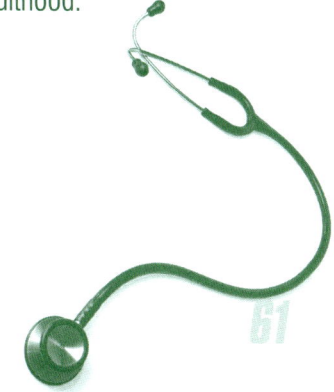

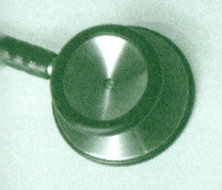

What's in a name?

'For decades, purveyors of fatty, sugary, salty foods have said, "There is no such thing as bad food, only bad diets." '

Professor Tim Lang

Kid Net

The food and drink manufacturers have devised a strategy for netting new customers.

Children with their own email addresses are encouraged to contact food companies direct. *Chewits*, *Frosties*, *Kinder Surprise*, *Nesquik*, *Panda Pops* and *Skittles* (among others) are printing codes on their packets which children must quote to get into the programmes. The code is just a 'one-off' so many purchases have to be made to keep regular contact.

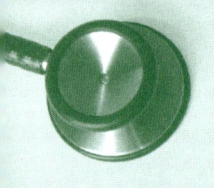

Sweet books

Companies such as Hershey in the US have published a number of primary school books, *Hershey's Kisses: Counting Board Book, The Hershey's Kisses Addition Book* and *The Hershey's Kisses Subtraction Book* in which all the material is depicted in terms of their own brand of chocolate bars.

Sweet hotline

British Telecom (BT) is planning to sell confectionery and fizzy drinks from their telephone kiosks to reverse the losses from 70,000 kiosks across the countryside. The BT sweet-talk may lure children away from their mobiles and give urgent calls new meaning!

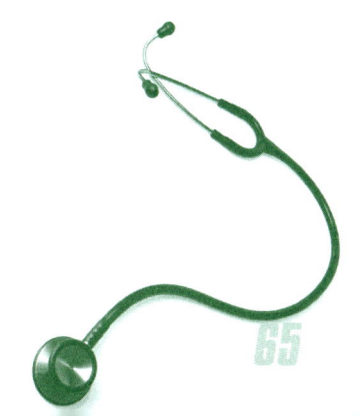

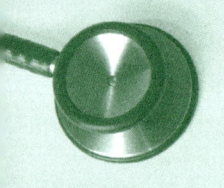

Unpalatable news

In spite of governments reminding us of the need to lower the intake of sugar, fat and salt, the fat in children's lunchboxes has increased by 3g over the past year. After sandwiches, crisps were found in 69% of lunchboxes, along with biscuits and chocolate bars (58% of lunchboxes), with cereal bars coming in at 29%.

Passing the orals

A Children's Dental Health survey, with a total of 12,698 schoolchildren aged 5, 8, 12 and 15 years, showed that children's permanent teeth are the best to date, with a decrease in plaque, gum and other oral conditions. There was a decline in decay, cavities and fillings (although those with fillings had multiple fillings).

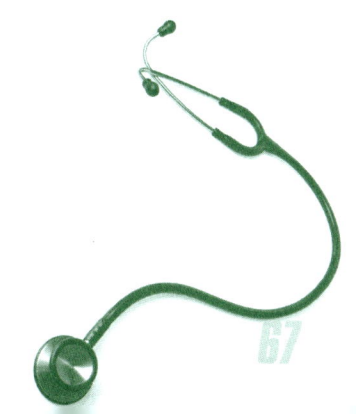

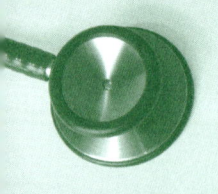

Thanks for the memory

'We can hear a melody for only a few seconds and yet carry it with us for a lifetime. Experience somehow leaves its mark on the mind. But how can something as fleeting as song take on substance and become part of the brain, part of the body?'

George Johnson

More than the sum of the parts

'Our memories are card-indexes consulted,
and then put back in disorder by
authorities whom we do not control.'
Cyril Connolly

'If the brain was so simple we could understand it,
we would be so simple that we couldn't.'
Lyall Watson

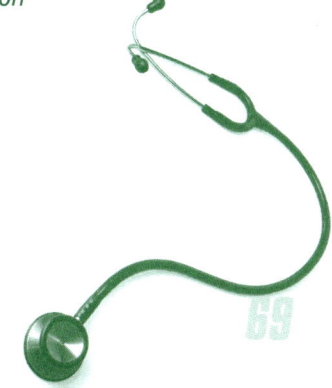

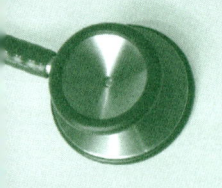

Aide-mémoire

'Education in general can bestow benefits on cognitive function in later life.'
Professor Clive Ballard

Language skills keep the brain sharper for longer. A Canadian study showed that bilingual participants responded faster across the age ranges represented and also showed a slower rate of decline for some of the processes associated with ageing.

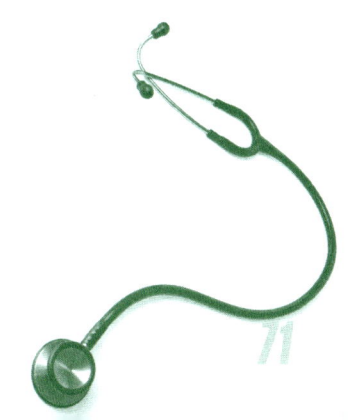

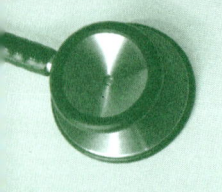

The delete key

Traumatic experiences wipe out memories including those associated with the trauma itself. While people will never forget the traumatic experience, they do not remember all the details, probably due to the high levels of *cortisol* and *adrenalin* released as a physical response to the stressful situation.

A head for heights

Scientists at the University of Florida have taught rat brain cells to fly a simulated F-22 jet!

Twenty-five thousand neural cells from a rat embryo were kept alive in a Petri dish. The cells were suspended in a special nurturing liquid and placed on a grid of 60 electrodes.

By manipulating the electrodes, the brain cells were taught to 'fly' the fighter plane.

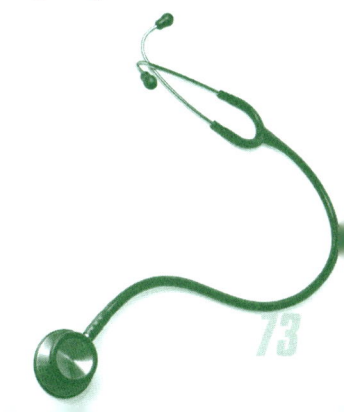

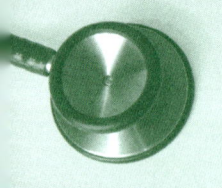

The night shift

Dreams are thought to be a dialogue between different parts of the brain exercised during the sleeping hours.

Waking experiences are too fast to process and are recorded for future analysis.

When we sleep the sorting process takes place, and the mind tries to make sense of it all.

Recorded dream material is scanned for similarities and patterns, matching new information with what is already known.

If there is no logical pathway between item A and item B, a bizarre link might emerge and be experienced as a nightmare.

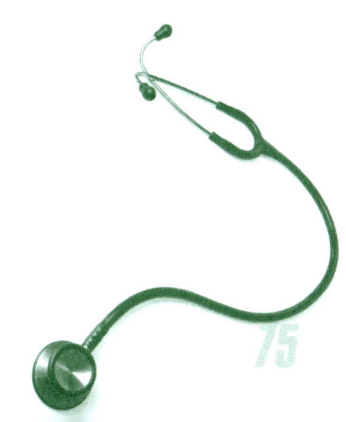

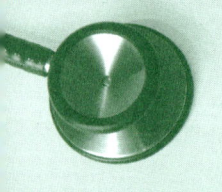

Stroke loss

A person suffering a stroke loses:
- 1.9 million brain cells;
- 14 billion synapses;
- 7.5 miles of nerve fibres each minute;
- 3.6 years of life for each hour of untreated oxygen-starved brain.

Combat stress

Combat stress is a recurring problem. Since the second Gulf War some 460 soldiers have been discharged with mental health problems, 50 being diagnosed with *Post Traumatic Stress Disorder (PTSD)*. Suicides following the war were five times higher than combat fatalities.

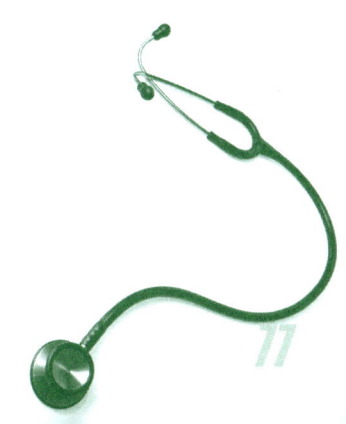

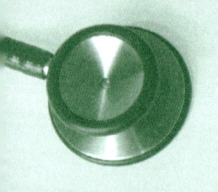

PTSD sufferers have: poor concentration, intense fear, insomnia and recurring, intrusive flashbacks to scenes better forgotten. Many drink to drown their sorrows, or find themselves in trouble through their eccentric or explosive behaviour. Currently, 5,000 ex-servicemen and women are imprisoned.

Stress less

'If you ask what is the single most important key to longevity, I would have to say it is avoiding worry, stress and tension. And if you didn't ask me, I'd still have to say it.'

George Burns

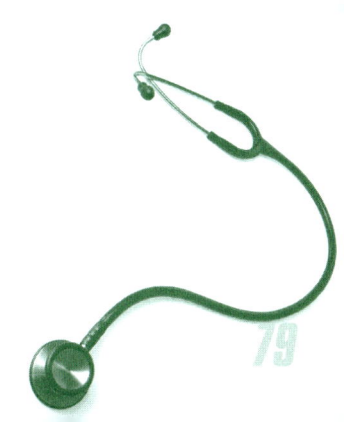

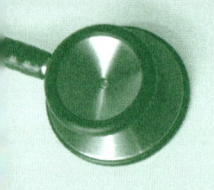

Busy doing nothing?

'Don't underestimate the value of Doing Nothing, of just going along, listening to all the things you can't hear, and not bothering.'

Pooh's Little Instruction Book,
inspired by A. A. Milne

Take time out

'A poor life this if, full of care,
We have no time to stand and stare.'
W. H. Davies

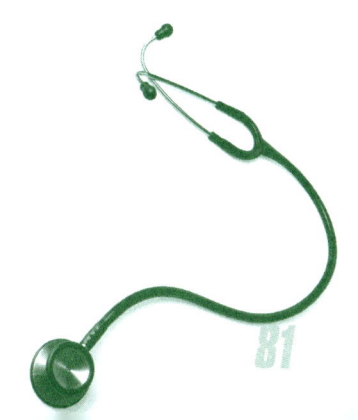

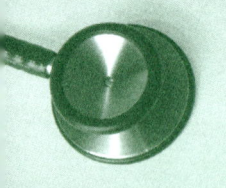

Don't catch cold!

'Pressure and stress is the common cold of the psyche.'
Andrew Denton

The responsible choice

'Stress is not what happens to us. It's our response TO what happens. And RESPONSE is something we can choose.'

Maureen Killoran

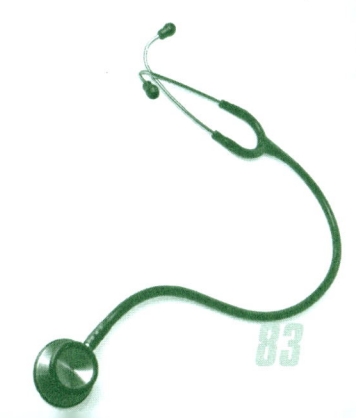

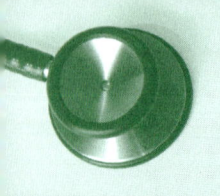

Sound advice

'Don't sweat the small stuff . . .
and it's all small stuff.'
Richard Carlson

Hippopota my goodness!

Scientists have discovered that hippopotamus sweat has a red and an orange pigment which may be useful to human health.

The red is a superior antibacterial which can speed skin healing, while the two can be used as an anti-UV screen to protect from over-exposure to the sun.

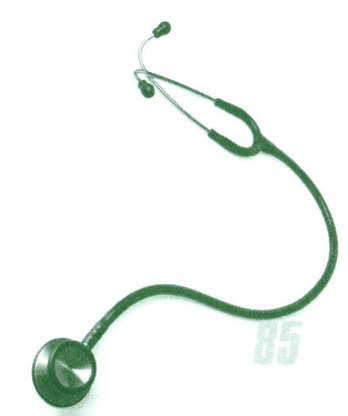

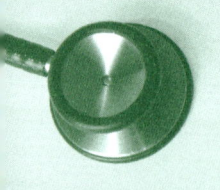

A frog in the throat

A man in the province of Hunan (China) whose doctor prescribed six raw frogs (yes, in the twenty-first century!) a day for his patient, who had neck ache, died after eating 130 of the frogs because they were infected with parasites.

It is not known exactly how even parasite-less frogs could have helped the man!

Something in the air

A German study showed that women living in the vicinity of toxic waste incinerators increased the chances of having twins.

Around 5% of mothers closest to the pollution had double the rate of twins of mothers further afield.

The downside to the study showed in low birth-weights, infant deaths and an increase in thyroid problems for the children.

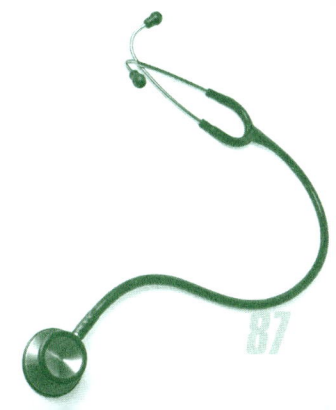

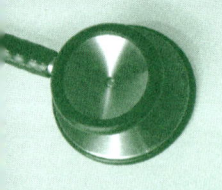

Bad air days

The need for a safe, effective and cheap anti-malarial drug is a vital necessity as around 300-500 million malarial treatments are needed annually.

One million children in Sub-Saharan Africa die of malaria each year – one about every thirty seconds. A three-day course of treatment should be sufficient to cure the malaria.

A hidden menace

Lloyds pharmacies introduced a free in-store glucose testing service and have screened 500,000 people for type 2 diabetes. About 72% of those referred to GPs had either type 2 or elevated blood glucose levels.

A Euro Heart Study found that 58% of 4,900 people with heart disease had diabetes but did not know it.

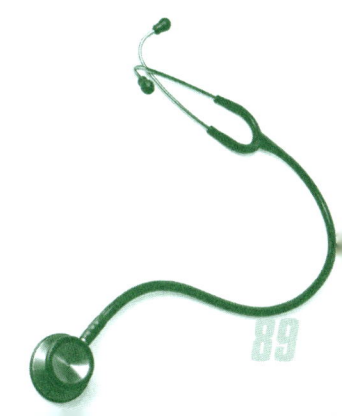

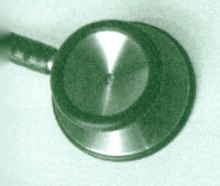

A glow in the dark?

Many are concerned that irradiated food might give them radiation sickness or the side effects associated with some cancer treatments.

There is no evidence of such and the nutritional values of the foods remain unchanged. There is in any case change in the nutritional status of foods undergoing any storage or cooking method.

Snail relief

The cone snail – *conus magus* – found in waters off the Philippines, has a venomous harpoon, the venom of which is now being used to replace morphine in sufferers with a low tolerance to opiates.

Prialt, made in Japan, shuts down pain pathways by interrupting signals to the brain. However, it can cause nausea, dizziness and blurred vision which some may consider a small price to pay for pain relief.

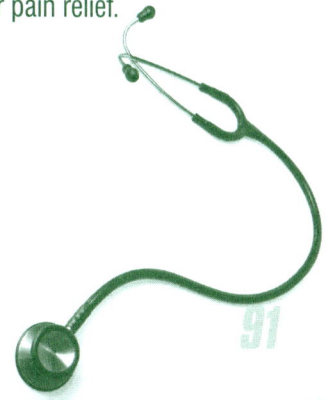

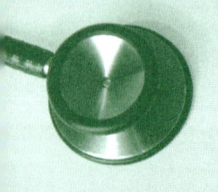

Doodlebugs

Streptococcus suis is a bacterial condition found in pigs in China. It has jumped species and caused ill health in 206 people, killing 38 and leaving 18 critically ill.

WHO's concern is that people will be affected by infected meat and develop meningitis-like symptoms, permanent hearing loss, arthritis or pneumonia.

Mind the gaps!

At an average speed of 65 mph
car telephone signals have:
- variations in sound quality
- 300 millisecond time-lags in conversation
- 300 millisecond breaks in signal quality every ten seconds

The brain has difficulty in piecing together the signals as coherent conversation and may distract the driver, thus contributing to an accident.

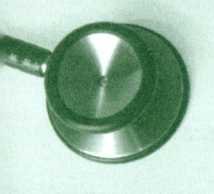

High noon

A US National Cancer Institute has shown that the incidence of colon, breast and prostate cancers are lower where sun-generated vitamin D is at its highest.

In the UK a prostatic cancer study found that men with the lowest lifetime exposure to the sun were three times more likely to be in the cancer group.

Sick buildings

'We now realise that how we design the built environment may hold tremendous potential for addressing many of the nation's greatest current public health concerns, including obesity, cardiovascular disease, diabetes, asthma, injury, depression, violence and social inequities.'

Dr Richard Jackson

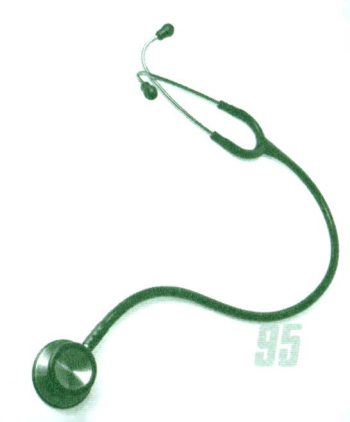

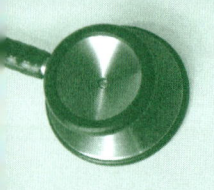

A 'reasonable' risk

Acceptable daily intakes (ADI) are arrived at by dividing the highest non-toxic animal dose by what is called an uncertainty/safety factor (100^2).

There are no means at present to assess the extent to which this factor is more than a 'guesstimate'.

PASSCLAIM

PASSCLAIM is an acronym for *Process for the Assessment of Scientific Support for Claims on Foods* and is the European underpinning for the regulatory bodies concerned with health-related functional foods.

These include: margarines to reduce cholesterol; yoghurts to provide right gut flora; *lycopene*-rich tomato products to reduce cancer risks; berry *flavanoids*, herbs and spices claiming to reduce a range of health complaints.

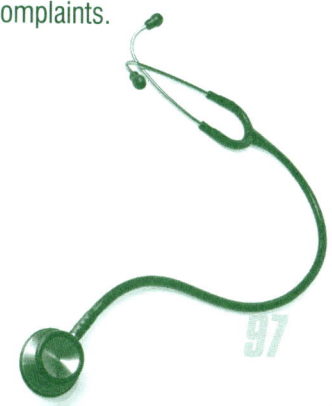

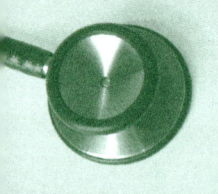

Sweet and sour

Between 1% and 10% of *Aspartame* users have reported acute adverse effects to the sweetener: severe headaches, blurred vision, and occasionally epileptic-type seizures.

A Washington University paper reported that *Aspartame* use had been responsible for a particular type of brain tumour called *glioblastoma*.

Loss of effect

Antivirals, antibiotics and antimicrobials have ever shorter lives as humans become resistant to their effects.

At the present time concerns have been expressed that *ciproflaxin*, used in the treatment of *campylobacter* in humans, is not effective in dealing with 19-40% of the strains clinically identified.

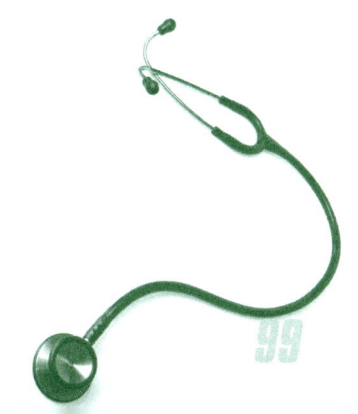

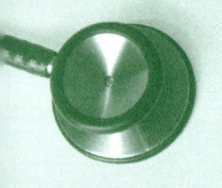

Pecking order

Factory farming techniques appear to increase the possibility of drug resistance. Tests on birds from organic farms and factory farms with chickens having *campylobacter* strains in their gut showed significant differences in antibiotic resistance – less than 2% for the former compared with anything from 46 to 47% in the latter.

Sexplosion

In the UK:
- there has been a 500% increase in *syphilis* over a decade;
- 1 in 10 of the population has experienced a sexually transmitted disease;
- *gonorrhoea* figures have doubled;
- 1 in 10 sexually active young people have *Chlamydia* (a micro-organism infecting the genital tract);
- about 41,500 people are living with *HIV/AIDS* (and around 30% are undiagnosed).

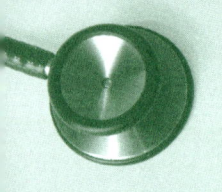

The food of love

'One of the prime causes of marital discord –
nutritional deficiency – is often overlooked. . . .
I have found that in a surprising number of
broken marriages, spouses suffered
from a blood sugar imbalance.

'Many of these husbands and wives showed symptoms of irritability, violent temper, abnormal sensitivity and extreme fatigue. In most cases there was no evidence of organic disease. Corrective nutritional guidance dispelled these unpleasant symptoms for many spouses – and, in the process, often bolstered crumbling marriages.'

Dr Cecilia Rosenfield

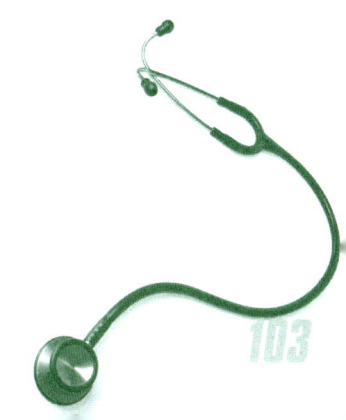

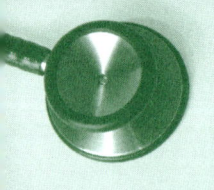

Somewhere to go!

'Lavatories date, in the UK, back to the Roman occupation. In 1423 the famous Dick Whittington (Lord Mayor of London) donated a toilet to the city in the form of a 'long house' having seating for 120 men and women.

The first flushing toilet was made for Queen Elizabeth 1 by Sir John Harrington, and the now familiar water closet (WC) was patented by Londoner Alexander Cummings in 1775.

The end is nigh!

Actuary researcher Francis Fernandes says: 'Society might dictate that life has to finish at a certain age regardless of health.' We can only hope that his statement is not connected to the 'Take a Loved One to a Doctor' day promoted by the American Public Health Association!

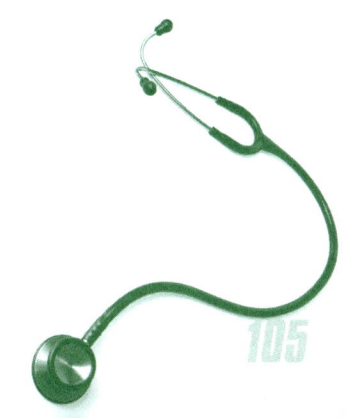

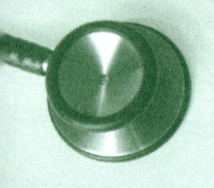

Star treatment

There is an irony in the fact that not only does the avian flu virus come from the East but also its remedy.

A rare herb grown in China – *star anise* (used as a flavouring in cooking) – produces *shikimic acid* from which *oseltamivir* or *Tamiflu* is made.

Bird flu

Migratory birds with the *H5N1* virus have devastated Asian poultry flocks and their Australian counterparts. Ducks migrating from southern China took the virus to Korea and Siberia. A related virus *H5N2* led to the cull of 30,000 ostriches in South Africa.

Fears that the virus may kill humans have been realised with the death of 24 people in Asia.

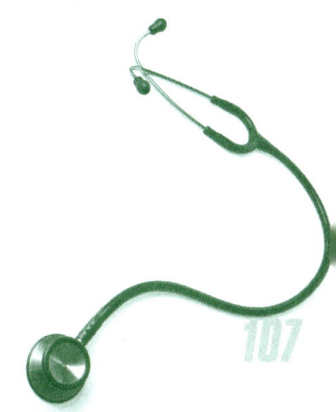

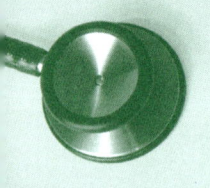

Hair today . . .

An EC watchdog is worried that some dark-coloured permanent hair dyes used frequently may cause cancer. The ingredients *paraphenylenediamine* and *tetrahydro-6-nitroquinoxaline* have been shown to damage genetic material and, in laboratory studies, have caused cancer in animals.

Un(der)armed

Studies in Britain have shown that traces of chemicals absorbed into the skin migrate to breast tissue, especially traces of chemicals called *parabens*.

A University of Reading study tested 20 different human breast tumours and found traces of *paraben* in each. Animal studies have show parabens to mimic the action of the hormone *oestrogen*.

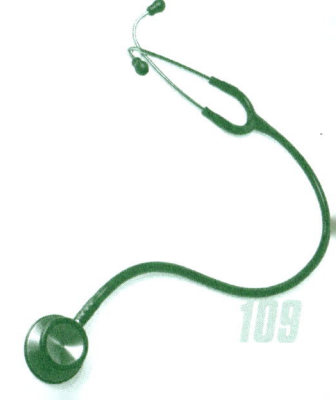

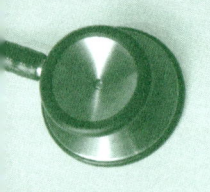

Bust-up!

A new Japanese chewing gum made from an extract of the plant *Pueraria mirifica* claims to help enhance the size, shape and tone of breasts due to the presence of *phytoestrogens* in the plant.

Called Bust-up gum, its wide-ranging claims need to be verified before causing any bust-ups worldwide and damaging credibility for health-related functional foods!

Eyes right!

A new craze in the Netherlands is to have minute jewellery embedded in the eyeball. Star- and heart-shaped pieces of platinum about a millimetre in size are adding sparkle to eyes.

The craze serves no medical purpose and has not undergone safety trials, so the long-term effects of the cosmetic application are not known.

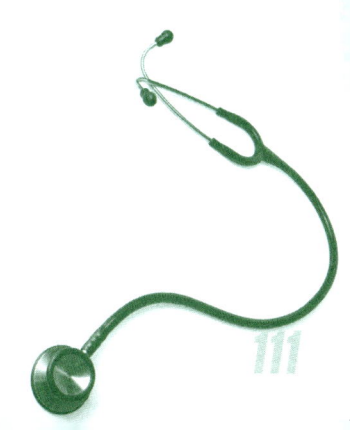

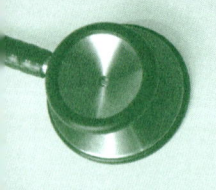

Watch-dog

Sony has made a robotic dog – *Aibo* – to help fight flab. It has four different behaviours that respond to a dieter's question, 'How am I doing?' and the dieter's compliance.

If the regime has been strictly adhered to, *Aibo* jumps up and down and wags its tail vigorously, plays vibrant music and flashes brightly-coloured LEDs all over the body. If the calorie intake has been too high, *Aibo* moves lethargically and plays low-energy music.

Keep within the limits

Dieting is the penalty for exceeding the feed limit.

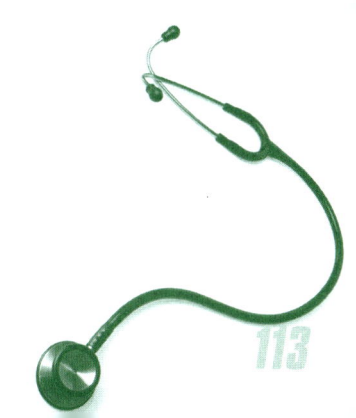

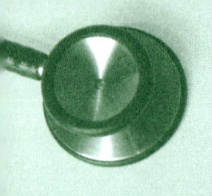

Over the border

'Move a little more and eat a little less.'

Dr Alan Maryon Davies

It is estimated that 90% of obesity (with its diabetes consequences) could be abolished by walking an extra 2,000 steps and reducing calorie intake by a mere 100 calories a day!

Mind what you eat!

'Indulgence of appetite is the greatest cause
of physical and mental debility and lies
at the foundation of the feebleness
which is apparent everywhere.'

Ellen White

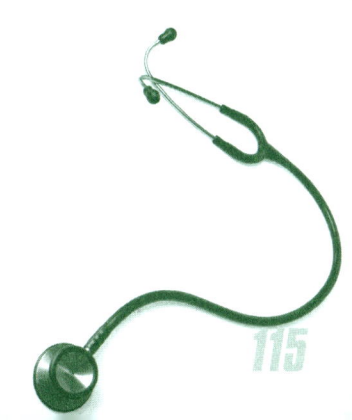

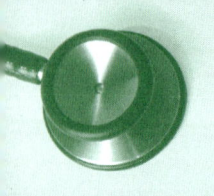

Cooking up trouble?

'Doctors are always working to preserve our health and cooks to destroy it, but the latter are the more often successful.'
Denis Diderot

Spud bashing!

Potatoes were introduced to the UK in the 1590s. The Protestants would not plant them because they were not mentioned in the Bible, and to get around this theological deficit, Irish Catholics sprinkled their seed potatoes with holy water and planted them on Good Friday!

The name *spud* was an Irish gift to the English language deriving from their word for the spade used to dig the potatoes.

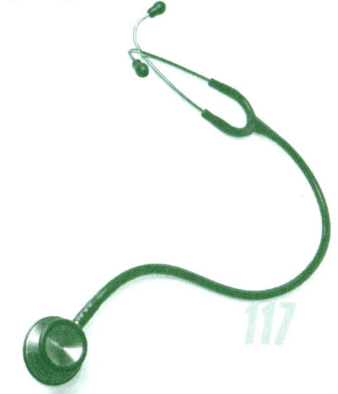

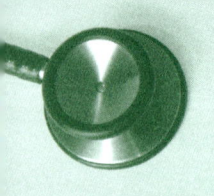

On your bike!

'This increasingly sedentary lifestyle is habitual, but it has also to do with our environment. For example, some parents do not believe it is safe to let their children play outside so instead they are watching television. Part of the solution, which requires partnership at all levels, could be to introduce things like safe play zones or set bicycle routes.'

Professor Siân Griffiths

When the velocipede and then the bicycle became popular the direst of consequences were anticipated: *kyphosis bicyclistarum* (cyclist's spine or cyclist's stoop); bicycle hernia; bicycle heart; cyclist's sore throat; the incessant tension of keeping the eye on the road; and cyclist's neurosis, to name a few.

Now cycling is a recognised and prescribed preventive or remedy. The wheels have turned!

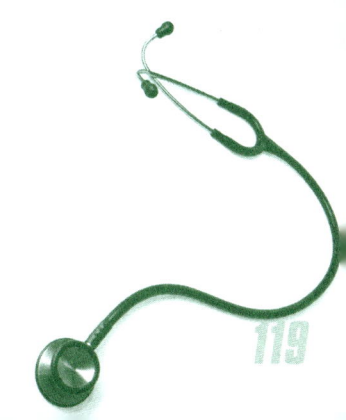

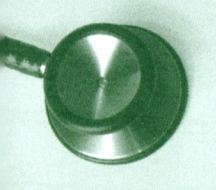

The best prescription

'The best six doctors anywhere
And no one can deny it
Are sunshine, water, rest, and air
Exercise and diet. . . .

'These six will gladly you attend
If only you are willing
Your mind they'll ease
Your will they'll mend
And charge you not a shilling.'
Nursery rhyme

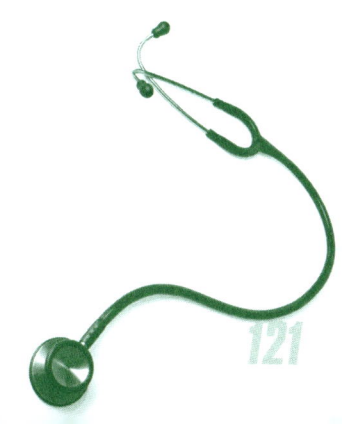

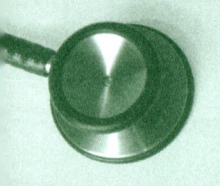

Full circle?

A Short History of Medicine – 2000BC.
'Here, eat this root.' – 1000BC.
'That root is heathen, say this prayer.' – AD1850.
'That prayer is superstition, drink this potion.'
– AD1940.
'That potion is snake oil, swallow this pill.'
– AD1985.
'That pill is ineffective, take this antibiotic.'
– AD2000.
'That antibiotic is artificial. Here, eat this root.'

Author unknown

The power of positive thinking

'To wish to be well is a part of becoming well.'
Seneca

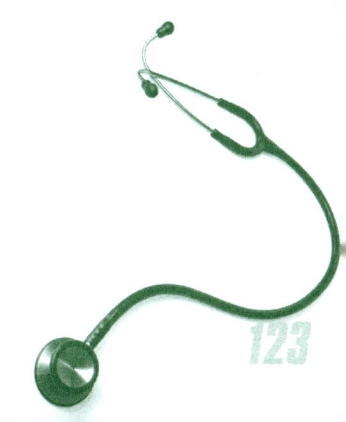

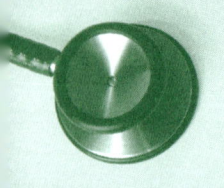

The whole = the sum of the parts

'The concept of total wellness recognises that our every thought, word, and behaviour affects our greater health and well-being. And we, in turn, are affected not only emotionally but also physically and spiritually.'

Greg Anderson

The heart of the matter

'The sincere acceptance of the principles and teachings of Christ with respect to the life of mental peace and joy, the life of unselfish thought and clean living, would at once wipe out more than half the difficulties, diseases and sorrows of the human race.'

Dr William Sadler

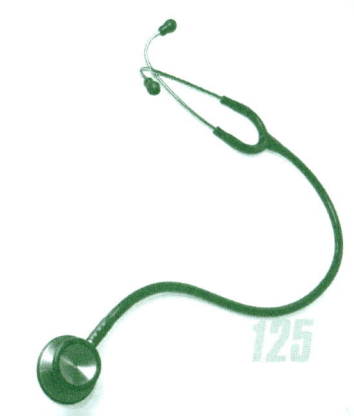

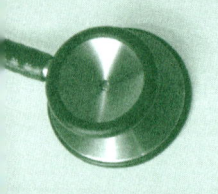

'Christ is the wellspring of life. That which many need is to have a clearer knowledge of Him; they need to be patiently and kindly, yet earnestly, taught how the whole being may be thrown open to the healing agencies of heaven. When the sunlight of God's love illuminates the darkened chambers of the soul, restless weariness and dissatisfaction will cease, and satisfying joys will give vigour to the mind and health and energy to the body.'

Ellen White

On the right track

'A person whose mind is quiet and satisfied in God is in the pathway to health.'
Ellen White

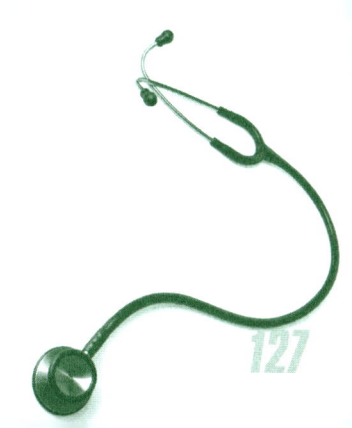

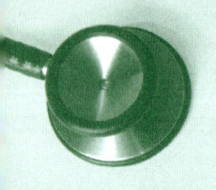

Be good to yourself

'Dear friend, I pray that you may enjoy good
health and that all may go well with you,
even as your soul is getting along well.'

3 John 2

'If you don't take care of yourself, the undertaker
will overtake that responsibility for you.'

Carrie Latet